YOUR KNOWLEDGE HAS VALUE

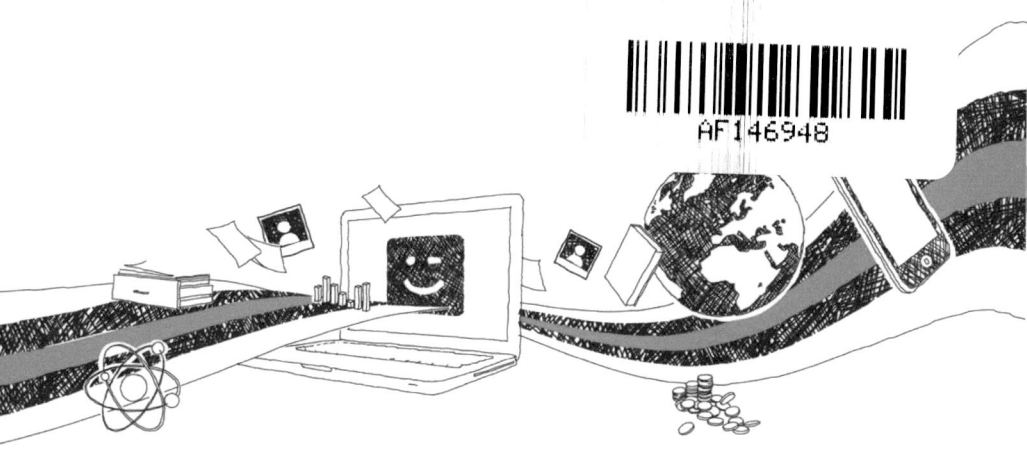

- We will publish your bachelor's and master's thesis, essays and papers

- Your own eBook and book - sold worldwide in all relevant shops

- Earn money with each sale

Upload your text at www.GRIN.com and publish for free

The Coronavirus. An infection prevention and control case study

John Die

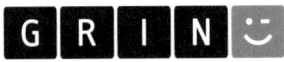

Bibliographic information published by the German National Library:

The German National Library lists this publication in the National Bibliography; detailed bibliographic data are available on the Internet at http://dnb.dnb.de.

ISBN: 9783346361059
This book is also available as an ebook.

© GRIN Publishing GmbH
Nymphenburger Straße 86
80636 München

All rights reserved

Print and binding: Books on Demand GmbH, Norderstedt, Germany
Printed on acid-free paper from responsible sources.

The present work has been carefully prepared. Nevertheless, authors and publishers do not incur liability for the correctness of information, notes, links and advice as well as any printing errors.

GRIN web shop: https://www.grin.com/document/992782

An infection prevention & control case study about a novel coronavirus (nSARS-CoV-2) spreading within the community

Townsville, 2020.

Table of content

Part A – Case Study 1
    Introduction 1
    Analysis of contributing factors 2
    Conclusion 5

Part B – Governance Report 6
    The Problem and its Impact 6
    Management of the Issues 6
        Hygiene concepts 6
        Staff education 7
    Future Prevention Strategies 8
    Expected Outcomes 8

References 10

Part A – Case Study

Introduction

A novel virus broke out in a in a city in southern China last year and developed to a major public health threat within a few months. The pandemic began with an outbreak of pneumonia with unknown origin (1) because of an infection of the lower respiratory tract (2). Soon, the novel pathogen was identified as a novel coronavirus, described as novel coronavirus pneumonia (NCP) by the Chinese government (2).

The family *Coronaviridae* is a monogeneric group of 11 viruses which infect vertebrates (3). *Coronaviridae* infect their hosts by horizontal transmission via the fecal/oral route (3). Three virus species are important for humans and are possible public health threats: SARS-CoV, which caused the Severe Acute Respiratory Syndrome (SARS) and was responsible for the pandemic in the years 2002 and 2003 (4), MERS-CoV, which caused the severe and fatal Middle East Respiratory Syndrome (MERS) and first occurred in the year 2012 (5), and SARS-CoV-2, which cause the Coronavirus Disease 2019 (COVID-19) and is responsible for the current pandemic. CoV is the abbreviation for Coronavirus. *Coronaviridae* are zoonotic pathogens with animal reservoirs. Their natural reservoirs are bats. It is very likely that the viruses crossed the species border from bats to humans. However, intermediate hosts could play an important role in transmission (6). As example, MERS-CoV can be found widely in dromedaries (7). In China, coronaviruses have been found in various species of horseshoe bats (*Rhinolophus spp.*), a genus of bats with 106 species that occurs in the complete Old World (Europe, Africa, Asia, Australia and Oceania) (6). The virus was identified by the Chinese Centers for Disease Control. It spread to the entire country within 30 days that showed the highly contagious nature of the pathogen (8). Due to this threat, China started strict infection prevention and control measures, including the complete lockdown of the Chinese city Wuhan, the greatest quarantine action in the modern world (9).

So far, possible animal reservoirs or intermediate hosts for SARS-CoV-2 are still unknown. After it was discovered in pangolins, several scientists hypothesized, that those animals could be a possible intermediate host (10, 11). It is likely, that the animal markets in Wuhan were the epicentres of the current pandemic. Night and wet markets are common in Asian countries. Those markets sell a lot of different goods, including meat, seafood and, (sometimes wild) animals (12). That makes those markets to ideal hotspots for zoonotic diseases. Many scientists recommended to stop the trade with pangolins and other wild animals (11). Other scientists recommended a complete shutdown of those markets (12). Research here is important, because the knowledge of potential animal reservoirs would help to create useful infection prevention measures. Those measures include One Health (the connection between human, veterinary and environmental health) approaches. We will discuss principles and actions to reduce the risk of infections in a laboratory and research institute background in the following section.

Analysis of contributing factors

Due to its high level of infectivity, healthcare practitioners and other people, who deal with the virus, need to exercise special caution. Because the outbreak developed quick to a pandemic, other people outside the traditional healthcare field are also affected. This particularly affects people who work internationally and consequently have to travel a lot, including pilots, logisticians, politicians and people from the travel industry, but also internationally active doctors and medical aid organizations. Those populations need to exercise special caution as well. The virus is spread by close contact with infected persons, close contact with droplets of infected persons (cough or sneezes) or by touching of equipment and surfaces contaminated by respiratory droplets. The best way to avoid infections is to perform social distancing. Social media platforms, like Instagram, helped to spread this knowledge by posting certain stickers and using certain hashtags (13). However, social media has also disadvantages during a pandemic. The platforms are a very easy way to spread fake-news and conspiracy theories. In our connected world, medical conspiracy theorists have long ceased to be individually isolated priests, but rather networked groupings that are of particular importance within infection control. With demonstrations, as is currently the case in Germany, those people can destroy months of quarantine and medical work in just a few days (14). It is not without reason that the WHO listed anti-vaxxers as one of the major threats to the medicine and people's health (15).

To avoid infections in laboratories, the staff should follow the following guideline:

- Use protection clothes: To avoid the spread of the virus, laboratory staff should wear protection clothes, including a lab coat, gloves, and a mouth protection or face mask to reduce the spread of oral droplets. A good lab coat should protect the wearer, his or her clothes and the complete arms down to the hands. It should be made out of thick tissue to protect against fire and flammable liquids and chemical. A lab coat should not leave the lab and should not cleaned in the normal laundry at home.

- Perform hand hygiene: Hand hygiene is a key concept in disease control. With clean hands, the staff do not spread infectious particles (such as by touching surfaces without hand cleaning). If hands are visible dirty, the staff should use water and soap and wash their hands up to 60 seconds. If the hands are not visible dirty, the staff should use alcohol-based handrubs. Their application is faster than the classic handwash with soap. The staff should use handrubs often (such as when they enter or leave the lab). While healthcare workers, who work with patients, should use special handrubs, laboratory staff can simply use ethanol, which should be in every lab. Ethanol can also apply on gloves and should be part of every lab.

- Educate staff about current hygiene plans: It is important to teach the staff about new and changing hygiene plans. If not, the staff is not able to follow new rules.

- Educate staff about biological safety: Laboratories are restricted to many peoples.

  To reduce the risk of spread, labs should only enter by educated staff. That includes safety briefings and other further instructions (such as fire safety and first aid). Higher secured labs need stricter and longer briefings. Staff with the authorization for lower security levels must not enter higher security level labs. However, the authorization for higher secured labs include the authorization for lower secured labs. Medical test could be mandatory for higher security levels. During this pandemic, it could make sense to make COVID-test and medical checks mandatory for laboratory staff and lower security levels. That includes also a mandatory vaccination.

- Frequent cleaning: Like hand cleaning, the lab cleaning is also very useful to avoid the spread. The cleaning staff should also be educated like the laboratory staff. The lab rubbish should be disposed separately and properly. That includes autoclavation of lab disposal, even if the garbage has not come into contact with infectious material. Chemicals should be disposed properly to avoid contamination. Bacterial cultures should be killed before disposal. Standard bleaching is a good choice for this.

- Workplace cleaning, good working ethic: Like the lab, the workplaces inside should Be cleaned after the experiments. The scientists should clean their places by themselves. The work surface should be cleaned with pure ethanol. This point includes also a general good working ethic. Part of this is for example the correct labelling of the used bottles and liquids. A good working ethic reduces risks and increased the safety, and also an increased safety reduced the risk spreading.

- Properly equipped labs: To allow good and safety work, the labs should be equipped properly. That includes ethanol, filled in handy wash bottles, an autoclave, and the ability to store chemicals and biological materials correctly. The equipment should be easy to reach and there should enough abilities to separate the rubbish correctly.

Conclusion

New and emerging infectious diseases are a serious threat to humanity. Often, there are no or only insufficient medications. For that reason, targeted preventive measures are necessary, for example keeping a distance and social distancing. Although these measures differ only to a limited extent in the various areas, health care facilities, hospitals, but also medical and biological laboratories must exercise special care. Because laboratories do not work with patients, they have a lower fluctuation of people in the building. That makes infection control measures easier than in hospitals. Laboratories are safe places with many security and hygiene rules. Of course, it is important that those rules were followed by the staff. For that reason, certain briefings should be compulsory during the pandemic. However, the development of new treatments and medicine is one of the best measures against the pandemic. A possible vaccine is here the most important measure.

Part B – Governance Report

The Problem and its Impact

In part A, we have discussed the outbreak of the novel Coronavirus (nSARS-CoV2) and some associated and relevant contribution factors. In this section, we discuss the management of associated issues with a governance background.

In the late 2019, a novel Coronavirus broke out in the southern Chinese city Wuhan (16). First described as a pneumonia with unknown origin (1), the virus was fast identified as a novel Coronavirus (2).

Its high infectivity makes early control and public health activities very important. Patients, infected with the novel Coronavirus are infectious two days before they develop the first symptoms. Compared with SARS-CoV-1 (pandemic in 2002/2003, the patients were maximal infectious one week after the first symptoms occurred), the new COVI-Disease is more infectious (17).

This high infectivity and the absence of symptoms make the handling of the disease very hard. In part A, some possible interventions and activities to handle the pandemic in a research institute were described. Now, it is important to develop possible approaches and management strategies, to realize those activities.

Management of the Issues

We have discussed possible management actions in section A. In this section, we now focus more precise on these actions. The outlined actions were: Use protection clothes; perform hand hygiene; educate staff about current hygiene plans; educate staff about biological safety; frequent cleaning; workplace cleaning, good working etc. and properly equipped labs. A correct management requires close cooperation between scientists and their labs, health care practitioners and politicians. The described actions can be divided in two main categories: Measures to create a hygiene concepts and education of the staff.

Hygiene concepts

One of the best ways to manage a potential threat in a laboratory background is to wear protection clothing. Those clothes include a lab coat, gloves, maybe goggles. During the current pandemic, face masks showed some protection for the public (18). However, their use is still controversial (19).

During the pandemic, many countries introduced an obligation to wear masks. The mask wearer protects others rather than himself. If enough people wear masks, a group protection is created. But enforcing a mask requirement could be challenging. Many countries introduced fines. For example, the fine in Berlin (Germany) is around 500€ (20). Australia, one the other hand, is the only country with a GDP over 1 trillion US$ without a mask obligation (21). Other useful actions are hygiene performance. The CDC points out, that hand hygiene in situations like eating, face touching or after using the restrooms is one of the major actions to reduce the spread (22).

During the pandemic, laboratories should introduce multiple and mandatory hygiene concepts. For example, hand hygiene after special situations (lunch break for example) could be mandatory. However, auditing and surveillance of this could be challenging. It is relatively easy to introduce compulsory lab coats and gloves. They are already part of related laws and just need to be actively implemented. But auditing and surveillance of mandatory hand washing is not only almost impossible but also ethically problematic. An obvious implementation of this obligation could be, for example, be the monitoring of the washrooms. However, it is questionable whether the employees will allow this. Here it is probably best to rely on the employee's personal responsibility. In general, hygiene plans are easier to manage. The laboratory could create special plans that employees must adhere to. For example, certain guidelines, such as keeping the workplace clean, could become mandatory in special situations (like the current pandemic). Specially trained staff are responsible for compliance with these guidelines. In addition, compliance is ensured through state controls. These are already mandatory, but should take place more frequently in special situations.

Staff education

Another point to provide infection security and correct issue management is the right staff education. Educated staff work more safely and confidently. This of course also has an impact on the safety in the laboratory. Compared with the hygiene concept, it is easier to audit and surveillance the education. The politic has also more influence here. Useful actions are the introductions of special staff educational courses, which are special related to the current pandemic or associated with more basic infection and pandemic control. The courses could be created by the ministry of health and provided online. Topics in these courses could include, for example, "genetic safety", "biological security" or "infection and control management". Furthermore, the specialists described in the previous section who are responsible for checking the hygiene concept should also receive special training. Further trainings in "corporate health management" are also interesting. The job of a corporate health manager is to monitor the health of employees and to improve it (if necessary) through measures. In order to motivate staff for further training and more work, these can be credited and counted as official further training. Staff with a bachelor´s degree, the successfully completed training courses could be credited towards a master´s degree, for example.

Future Prevention Strategies

With a view on the climate change and other great changes, it is very likely that pandemics, like the current one, become more frequent in the future. In the past, health was just the absence of a disease. But today we know what health is influenced by many factors. Health is influenced by many different social determinants. For example, stress, social identity and socioeconomic status. Those determinants are called social determinants of health (23). The term was introduced by the British epidemiologist Michael Marmot (24). Vulnerable groups are particularly affected by pandemics. The current COVID-19 pandemic is no exception (25). Vulnerable groups are people in poor and developing countries, indigenous people, old and very young people and more. We must set a special focus on these groups to protect them during future outbreaks. For that reason, the United Nations created the Sustainable Development Goals. The Sustainable Development Goals are 17 goals of a global blueprint to achieve better health but also a better and more sustainable future for all. Relevant goals are No Poverty (Goal 1), Zero Hunger (Goal 2), Good Health and Well-Being (Goal 3), Clean Water and Sanitation (Goal 6) or Reduce Inequalities (Goal 10). The UN aims to achieve the goals by 2030 (26). Another example for the reduction of health inequities is the Australian Closing-the-Gap Campaign. The aim of the campaign, which was introduced in 2008, is to close the health gap between the Australian Indigenous population (Aboriginal and Torres Strait Islander People) and the other population. Life expectancy, education and health overall is still lower in Indigenous people (27). New Zealand has a similar policy. Those campaigns are just two examples how close cooperation between states, NGOs and researchers should be. The most important point is, that the great changes in the near future (the climate changes is the best example) requires close interactions from state to state.

Expected Outcomes

If all described measures are carried out correctly, the risk of infection in laboratories and similar facilities can be reduced. However, compared to other health care facilities (for example hospitals), laboratories have a clear advantage. On the one hand, laboratories are already designed as standard to keep the risk of infections as low as possible. It is also helpful that unlike medical institutions, laboratories do not work with patients. However, there are also disadvantages in laboratories that could be reduced by good and, above all, transparent management. Unlike hospitals, laboratories are only accessible to the public to a limited extent or not at all. This limitation increases with the risk of the pathogens being researched. As a result, laboratories and other scientific institutes, high-security laboratories in particular, are targeted victims of conspiracy theories. This was particularly evident in the current pandemic.

This development has gone so far that the WHO already speaks of an "infodemic" (28). Transparent management and disease control actions could be helpful and counteract this development. However, this is just a hypothesis. In the end, however, it is already helpful if the infection is contained. Even the smallest of measures is helpful during a global pandemic.

References

1. Esakandari H, Nabi-Afjadi M, Fakkari-Afjadi J, Farahmandian N, Miresmaeili SM, Bahreini E. A comprehensive review of COVID-19 characteristics. *Biol Proced Online* 2020;22:19.

    https://doi.org/10.1186/s12575-020-00128-2.

2. Yuen KS, Ye ZW, Fung SY, Chen CP, Jin DY. SARS-CoV-2 and COVID-19: The most important research questions. *Cell Biosci* 2020;10:40.

    https://doi.org/10.1186/s13578-020-00404-4.

3. Siddell SG, Anderson R, Cavanagh D, Fujiwara K, Klenk HD, Macnaughton MR, Pensaert M, Stohlman SA, Sturman L, van der Zeijst BA. Coronaviridae. *Intervirology* 1983;20(4):181-189.

    https://doi.org/10.1159/000149390.

4. Anderson RM, Frazer C, Ghani AC, Donnelly CA, Riley S, Ferguson NM, Leung GM, Lam TH, Hedley AJ. Epidemiology, transmission dynamics and control of SARS: the 2002-2003 epidemic. *Philos Trans R Soc Lond B Biol Sci* 2004;359(1447):1091-1105.

    https://doi.org/10.1098/rstb.2004.1490.

5. Machkay IM, Arden KE. MERS coronavirus: diagnostic, epidemiology and transmission. *Virol J* 2015;12:222.

    https://doi.org/10.1186/s12985-015-0439-5.

6. Hu B, Ge X, Wang LF, Shi Z. Bat origin of human coronaviruses. *Virol J* 2015;12:221.

    https://doi.org/10.1186/s12985-015-0422-1.

7. Zumla A, Hui DS, Perlman S. Middle east respiratory syndrome. *Lancet* 2015;386(9997):995-1007.

    https://doi.org/10.1016/S0140-6736(15)60454-8.

8. The Novel Coronavirus Pneumonia Emergency Response Epidemiology Team. The epidemiological characteristics of an outbreak of 2019 novel coronavirus disease (COVID-19) – China, 2020. *China CDC Weekly* 2020;2(8):113-122.

    https://doi.org/10.46234/ccdcw2020.032.

9. Graham-Harrison E, Kuo L. China´s coronavirus lockdown strategy: brutal but effective. *The Guardian*. Published March 20, 2020. Accessed August 18, 2020.

    https://www.theguardian.com/world/2020/mar/19/chinas-coronavirus-lockdown-strategy-brutal-but-effective.

10. Zhai SL, Wie WK, Lv DH, Xu ZH, Chen QL, Sun MF, Li F, Wang D. Where did SARS-CoV-2 come from? *Vet Rec* 2020;186(8):254.

    https://doi.org/10.1136/vr.m740.

11. Lam TTY, Jia N, Zhang YW, Shum MHH, Jiang JF, Zhu HC, Tong YG, Shi YX, Ni XB, Liao YS, Li WJ, Jiang BG, Wei W, Yuan TT, Zheng K, Cui XM, Li J, Pei GQ, Qiang X, Cheung WYM, Li LF, Sun FF, Qin S, Huang JC, Leung GM, Holmes EC, Hu YL, Guan Y, Cao WC. Identifying SARS-CoV-2-related coronaviruses in Malayan pangolins. *Nature* 2020;583(7815):282-285.

    https://doi.org/10.1038/s41586-020-2169-0.

12. Petrikova I, Cole J, Farlow A. COVID-19, wet markets, and planetary health. *Lancet Planet Health* 2020;4(6):e213-e214.

    https://doi.org/10.1016/S2542-5196(20)30122-4.

13. Hutchinson A. Instagram launches ´Stay Home´ sticker and story to encourage social distancing amid COVID-19 outbreak. *SocialMediaToday*. Published March 21, 2020. Accessed August 18, 2020.

    https://www.socialmediatoday.com/news/instagram-launches-stay-home-sticker-and-story-to-encourage-social-distan/574628/.

14. Leber S. Attila Hildmann gibt Juden die Schuld – und verteidigt Hitler. *Der Tagesspiegel*. Published June 19, 2020. Accessed August 18, 2020.

    https://www.tagesspiegel.de/themen/reportage/antisemitismus-im-netz-attila-hildmann-gibt-juden-die-schuld-und-verteidigt-hitler/25930880.html.

15. WHO. Ten threats to global health in 2019. *World Health Organization*. Published 2019. Accessed August 18, 2020.

    https://www.who.int/news-room/feature-stories/ten-threats-to-global-health-in-2019.

16. Seidel J. Mystery lab next to coronavirus epicentre. *news.com.au*. Published January 29, 2020. Accessed August 31, 2020.

    https://www.news.com.au/lifestyle/health/health-problems/mystery-lab-next-to-coronavirus-epicentre/news-story/3e5a32fe77263fe8ca81b091cc8d9c42.

17. Müller T. COVID-19-Patienten schon zweieinhalb Tage vor Symptombeginn infektiös. *Pneumo News* 2020;12(3):27-28.

    https://doi.org/10.1007/s15033-020-1826-1.

18. Beeson S, Behary N, Perwuelz A. Universal masking during COVID-19 pandemic: can textile engineering help public health? Narrative review of the evidence. *Prev Med* 2020;139:106236.

    https://doi.org/10.1016/j.ypmed.2020.106236.

19. Merkur.de. Coronavirus-Maßnahmen: WHO ändert Empfehlung zum Tragen von Masken. *Merkur*. Updated June 09, 2020. Accessed September 07, 2020.

    https://www.merkur.de/welt/coronavirus-deutschland-maskenpflicht-masken-bundeslaender-who-empfehlung-regeln-news-zr-13716654.html.

20. Wehner M. Wie Berlin gegen Maskenmuffel vorgeht. *Frankfurter Allgemeine*. Updated June 24, 2020. Accessed September 07, 2020.

https://www.faz.net/aktuell/politik/inland/wie-berlin-die-maskenpflicht-durchsetzt-bussgeld-bis-500-euro-16830422.html

21. Howard J, Talley N. Why are masks not yet mandatory in Australia? *The Sydney Morning Herald*. Published July 08, 2020. Accessed September 07, 2020.

    https://www.smh.com.au/national/why-are-masks-not-yet-mandatory-in-australia.20200708-p55a4k.html

22. National Center for Immunization and Respiratory Diseases (NCIRD), Division of Viral Diseases. How to protect yourself & others. *Centers for Disease Control and Prevention*. Updated July 31, 2020. Accessed September 07, 2020.

    https://www.cdc.gov/coronavirus/2019-ncov/prevent-getting-sick/prevention.html

23. Haslam C, Haslam SA, Jetten J, Cruwys T, Steffens NK. Life change, social identity, and health. *Annu Rev Psychol* 2020.

    https://doi.org/10.1146/annurev-psych-060120-111721

24. Marmot M. Michael Marmot: Evidence based optimist. *BMJ* 2015;351:h4577.

    https://doi.org/10.1136/bmj.h4577

25. Marmot M, Allen J. COVID-19: exposing and amplifying inequalities. *J Epidemiol Community Health* 2020;74(9):681-682.

    https://doi.org/10.1136/jech-2020-214720

26. Sustainable Development Goals. About the sustainable development goals. *United Nations*. No publication date. Accessed September 07, 2020.

    https://www.un.org/sustainabledevelopment/sustainable-development-goals/

27. National Indigenous Australian Agency. Closing the gap. *Australian Government*. Updated 2020. Accessed September 07, 2020.

    https://ctgreport.niaa.gov.au/

28. Caulfield T. Pseudoscience and COVID-19 – we´ve had enough already. *Nature* 2020.

    https://doi.org/10.1038/d41586-020-01266-z

YOUR KNOWLEDGE HAS VALUE

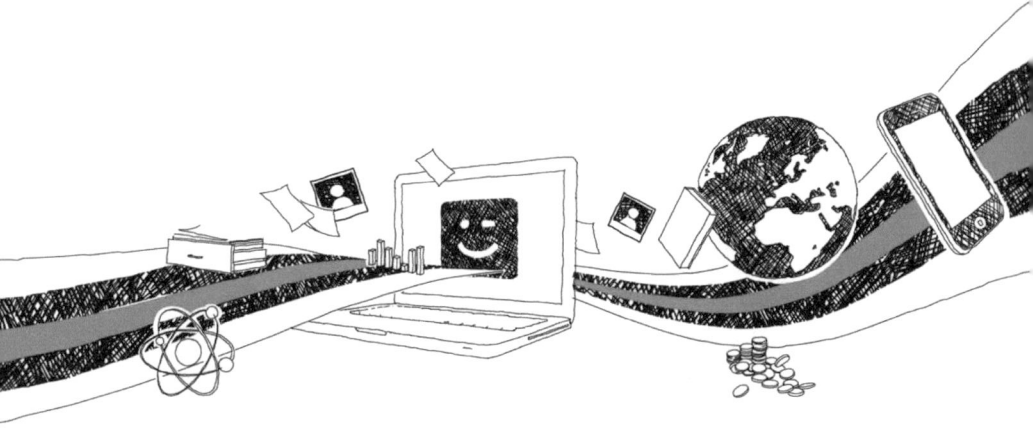

- We will publish your bachelor's and master's thesis, essays and papers

- Your own eBook and book - sold worldwide in all relevant shops

- Earn money with each sale

Upload your text at www.GRIN.com and publish for free

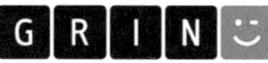